How to Get Rid of Asthma Naturally

By M. Usman

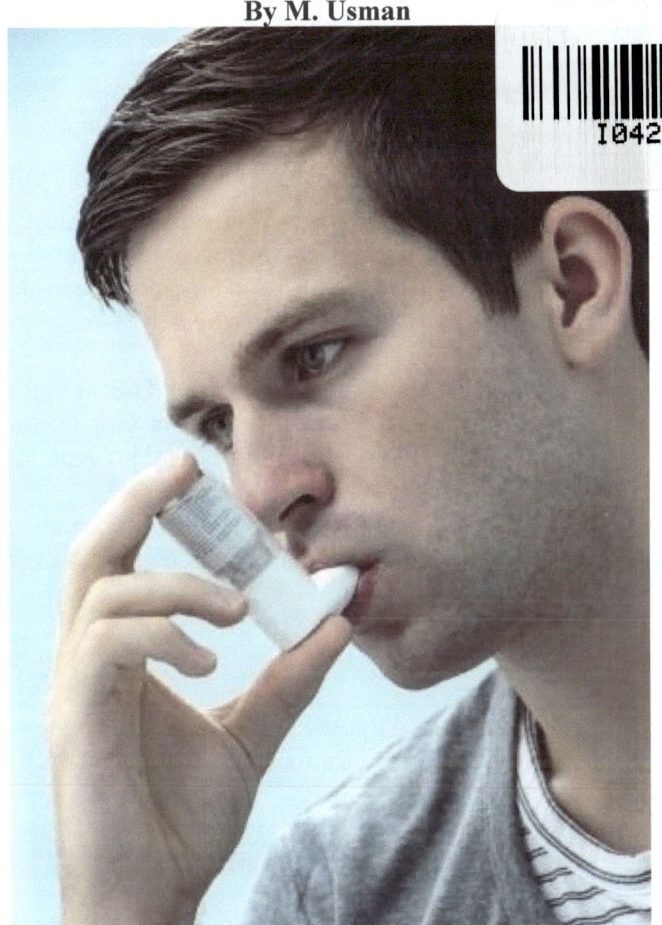

Health Learning Series

Mendon Cottage Books

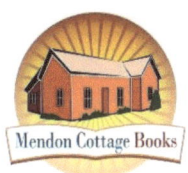

JD-Biz Publishing

Disclaimer

The information is this book is provided for informational purposes only. It is not intended to be used and medical advice or a substitute for proper medical treatment by a qualified health care provider. The information is believed to be accurate as presented based on research by the author.

The contents have not been evaluated by the U.S. Food and Drug Administration or any other Government or Health Organization and the contents in this book are not to be used to treat cure or prevent disease.

The author or publisher are not responsible for the use or safety of any diet, procedure or treatment mentioned in this book. The author or publisher is not responsible for errors or omissions that may exist.

Warning

The Book is for informational purposes only and before taking on any diet, treatment or medical procedure it is recommended to consult with your primary care provider.

Our books are available at

1. Amazon.com

2. Barnes and Noble

3. Itunes

4. Kobo

5. Smashwords

6. Google Play Books

Table of Contents

Introduction

"An estimated 22 million Americans have asthma; 6.5 million are under 18" (American College of Allergy, Asthma & Immunology)

Asthma is a serious complication of respiratory track which causes symptoms like chest congestion, coughing and difficulty in breathing.

"In America alone, asthma causes 4,000 deaths per year." (American College of Allergy, Asthma & Immunology)

Environmental pollution and too much exposure to harmful chemicals have significantly increased the susceptibility of people getting asthma. The death toll is expected rise even further. The cost of treatment of asthma is increasing. Accept it- No one likes going to a doctor. A single visit to a doctor costs too much.

"Americans spend, through direct and indirect expenses, a total of $19.7 million each year for the treatment of asthma." (American College of Allergy, Asthma & Immunology)

This book focuses on describing all the possible natural treatments of asthma. You don't have to go to great lengths to cure asthma. Sometimes, simple things in your cupboard or refrigerator can serve as homemade remedies for asthma. Another natural way is to treat asthma with herbs. Herbs are being used for the treatment of several ailments for thousands of years. But, it's an astounding fact that people consider them unsafe and difficult to use. Several experimentations have proved that herbs can cure several health conditions with virtually zero side effects. A simple change in life style can also help in curing asthma. Asthmatic attacks, in some cases, are triggered by eating certain food substances. So, having knowledge of what to eat and what to skip can actually decrease the frequency of asthmatic attacks.

Section one - Asthma – an overview

Asthma – What is Asthma?

Asthma is a common health condition related to an immune reaction taking place in the respiratory track. It's a breathing disorder characterized by several symptoms like air way obstruction, difficulty in breathing, tightness of chest, coughing and wheezing. For most of the people asthma is not a big problem. But, in reality it can cause serious hindrance in performing routine activities. If it goes untreated, it can produce serious and life threatening conditions.

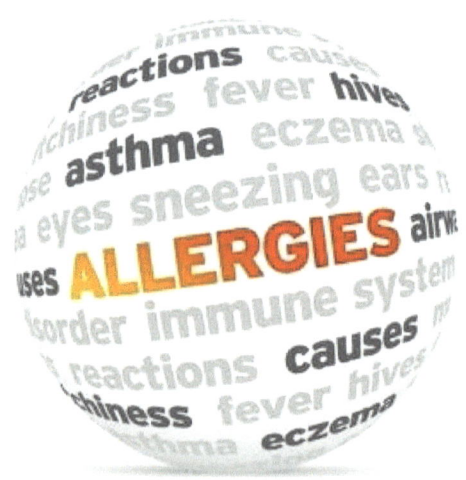

Asthma is an immune reaction triggered when the respiratory track is exposed to certain irritating stimuli. Human body has got a strong immune system which protects it from the harmful effects of foreign substances like chemicals, pollutants and organisms like bacteria and viruses. An important component of this immune system is "mast cells". These cells respond to the presence of certain "antigens" and release several mediators of inflammation, in the presence of these antigens. For example, if these cells are exposed to the smoke of cigarette, they'll release several chemicals which, in turn, will start a cascade of events leading to the development of symptoms of inflammation. These mediators cause spasm in the muscles of respiratory track, increase the production of mucus and make the respiration difficult.

Asthma is a combination of several environmental and genetic factors. The variability of these factors influences the severity of attacks and determines the responsiveness to therapy. There are several factors which are thought to cause asthma. Some of such factors are given below:

Environmental factors:

Several environmental factors are associated with the development of asthma. Such factors include:

- o Breathing in low quality air having high levels of pollutants like smoke, smog, fog and ozone.
- o Several house hold products, like detergents, soaps, skin care products etc, contain several chemicals which can trigger an intense asthmatic attack. Such products include chemicals like formaldehyde, phosphates etc.
- o House hold fungus, found on dish wash basins, washrooms, carpets etc, can also trigger such attack.
- o Several insects, like cockroaches and mites, can cause asthma.
- o Smoking is the most important cause of asthma in people of all age groups. Not only the active smokers but also the

passive smokers i.e. people exposed to the smoke of cigarette, are at high risk of development of asthma.

Hygiene hypothesis:

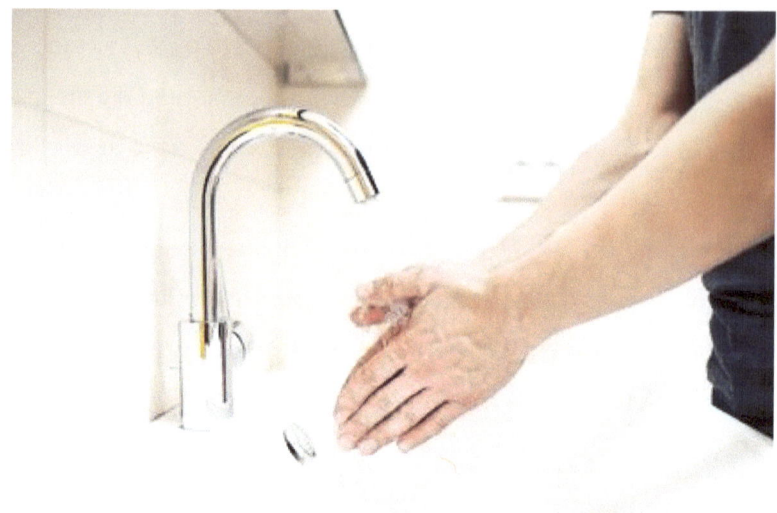

This hypothesis is exactly opposite to what one would expect. According to this hypothesis increased rates of asthma, worldwide, is due to excessive cleanliness and small sized families. This way the children and adults are less exposed to non-pathogenic bacteria and viruses. Exposure to such bacteria and viruses develops immunity against several diseases- asthma is one of such diseases. This mechanism is same as the process of vaccination in which non-virulent and non-pathogenic viruses and bacteria are inserted in the body to develop immunity against the virulent strains of bacteria and viruses. This hypothesis is supported by the fact that individuals living in farms or having pets are less prone to the development of asthma.

But, it's a well accepted fact that too much exposure to bacteria, viruses, dust, pollutants, smoke and insects can actually worsen the condition.

Genetic factors:

Genetic factors are one of the most important causes of asthma. This disease mostly runs in families. Several genetic factors contribute the development of asthma, like:

- o If one identical twin has asthma, the chances of the other having this disease are 25%.
- o Until now, 100 genes have been identified, mutation in which can lead to the development of asthma.

Medical conditions:

There is a strong link between certain medical conditions and asthma.

- o Obese people are more to the development of asthma.
- o People suffering from atopic dermatitis also show symptoms of asthma.
- o Chrug-Struss syndrome increases the chances of development of this immune disease.
- o This disease is also seen in people suffering from vasculitis i.e. inflammation of blood vessels.
- o Use of different medicines can develop asthma like symptoms. Such medicines include beta blockers, non-steroidal anti-inflammatory drugs (NSAIDs) and ACE inhibitors.

Symptoms – When you know it's coming…

There are several symptoms of asthma. The frequency, intensity and recurrence of these symptoms vary from person to person. The intensity of these symptoms also vary during different time of the day e.g. the attacks of asthma are very strong during late nights and are less strong during day time. Following are the major symptoms of asthma:

- Wheezing.
- Shortness of breath.
- Congestion of chest.
- Difficulty in breathing.
- Coughing.
- Sputum is frequently produced which is usually difficult to expel. The color of the sputum changes to "pus like" while recovering from the attack.
- Difficulty in sleeping or waking at once due to difficulty in breathing.
- Sneezing.

Aggravating factors:

Several conditions can worsen the symptoms of asthma.

- The symptoms of asthma usually aggravate when a person inhales cold and dry air.
- In some people, the symptoms of asthma worsen during exercise.
- In some cases, the symptoms of asthma exacerbate during night time. Body makes steroids, the levels of which alter during different time of the day. The level of these steroids is highest

during day time and lowest during night time. Steroids decrease inflammation and suppress the symptoms of asthma. That's why, the attacks of asthma are more intense and more frequent during night time.

o   The occurrence of asthma is mostly seen in individuals associated with certain occupation. Individuals working in plastic, paint, cigarette etc. industries are the highest risk.

o   In some individuals, eating certain food substance worsen the conditions.

Risk factors and complications– Why you should bother trying to avoid asthma?

Risk factors:

There are several factors which can increase the chances of you getting this disease. Such factors include:

- You're at a greater of development of asthma if your blood relatives i.e. immediate family members such as sibling and parents, have this condition.
- You're at greater risk if you've other allergic disease as well. There's a classical triad of atopic dermatitis, allergic rhinitis and asthma.
- Obesity is one of the most important risk factors for the development of asthma.
- Smokers, both active and passive smokers, are at highest risk to get this disease.
- If a female smokes during pregnancy then there's a high chance that her child will suffer from asthma.
- Exposure to exhaust fumes, both industrial and from vehicles, increase the chances of a person catching this disease.
- Exposure to chemicals like phosphates, PVC etc. is the greatest risk factor for asthma.
- Children having low weight at the time of birth are at the highest risk of development of asthma. Low birth weight indicates that the child has some kind of developmental abnormality. The development of lungs and respiratory track is usually impaired in such children. Poorly developed lungs, when exposed to environmental triggers, can develop a lethal asthmatic attack.

Complications:

Asthma can seriously affect the quality of life and can interfere with the routine activities of an individual. Complications of asthma include:

- The symptoms of asthma interfere with sleep, recreational activities and work.
- Poor performance at work or school during sick days.
- Chronic asthma can lead to the permanent narrowing of respiratory passage, which can lead to difficulty in breathing.
- Severe cases might need hospitalization.
- If you are on anti-asthma medications, you've to face several side effects of these medicines.

Section Two- Reducing Asthma.

Natural remedies – Who needs a doctor?

Asthma can be treated by the use of both medicines and natural remedies. Natural remedies have got an upper hand over allopathic medicines as they can suppress the symptoms of asthma with minimum, or virtually zero, side effects. These natural remedies focus on soothing the respiratory track and washing the mediators of inflammation. All such remedies are extremely cost effective and don't cost as much as the visits to your doctor. Moreover, the use of these remedies is very easy and you don't need any special technique or training, as required in the use of inhalers, to use these remedies. These remedies are easy to find and you don't have to go to great lengths to acquire these remedies. Above all, all these remedies naturally suppress the symptoms of asthma without causing serious side effects, as seen with the use of the most anti-asthma medicines. Natural remedies for asthma include:

- Homemade remedies are one of the most effective natural remedy for the treatment of asthma. These remedies come straight from your cupboard or refrigerator.
- Herbal remedies are being used for centuries for the treatment of several ailments. But it's an astounding fact that herbal method hasn't got as much acceptance as the modern treatment methods. People believe that herbs are unsafe and are injurious to health. Modern experiments have proven that herbal method is safe, easy to use, effective and has got minimal side effects.

- One of the most important trigger of an asthmatic attack is the use of certain type of food stuff. Certain foods contain proteins which act as "antigen trigger" for mast cells. For example some people are allergic to peanut butter. So, having knowledge of what to eat and what to skip can help a lot in curing asthma.
- In some cases, simple life style changes, such as regular exercise and abstinence from smoking, can help a lot in decreasing the frequency and intensity of asthmatic attacks.

Try some homemade remedies.

Luckily, a lot of homemade remedies are available which provide an effective cure from asthma. Such remedies include:

Normal saline solution:

It's one of the most effective homemade remedies for asthma. Saline solution is easily available in medical stores. A variety of preparations, like nasal drops or nasal sprays, are available in market. It helps get rid of asthma because of following basic reasons:

- Spraying or washing your nose helps clear the irritant stuck in the respiratory track.
- Second, it helps clear the mast cells and mediators of inflammation released by them.
- Saline solution has a soothing effect in general.

Honey:

Honey is used for the treatment of variety of ailments- asthma is one of such conditions. Honey reduces the soreness when used during throat infections. Honey is particularly very effective in the treatment of asthma. Honey contains a small amount of "pollen", which bees collect from different flowers. When this pollen is ingested, it produces anti bodies by triggering the immune system. But, the anti-bodies produced this way are not enough to develop obvious symptoms of inflammation. However, if such person is exposed to the triggers of asthma, like smoke or pollen, these anti-bodies eliminate such substances before they can initiate the symptoms of asthma.

Honey can be used in a variety of ways:

- You can 1-2 tea spoons of honey in a cup of water and heat it till it becomes Luke warm. Drink this water 1-2 times each day.
- You can add honey in your drinks and teas.
- You can add honey in your salads, meals and breakfast cereals.

Apple cider vinegar:

Apple cider vinegar is very effective for the treatment of asthma. It helps get rid of asthma because of following basic reasons:

- The obstruction of air passage during asthma is caused by the increase in the amount of mucous. This mucous causes symptoms like sneeze and cough. Apple cider vinegar decreases the production of mucous during asthma.
- It helps strengthen the lymphatic system of body. Lymphatic system is an essential part of defense mechanism of human body. It helps wash away the foreign particles like pollen or dust particles.

Quercetin:

It's a natural substance present in food stuff like broccoli and citrus food. It's a natural bioflavonoid which is very effective in reducing

Go green, Go for herbs.

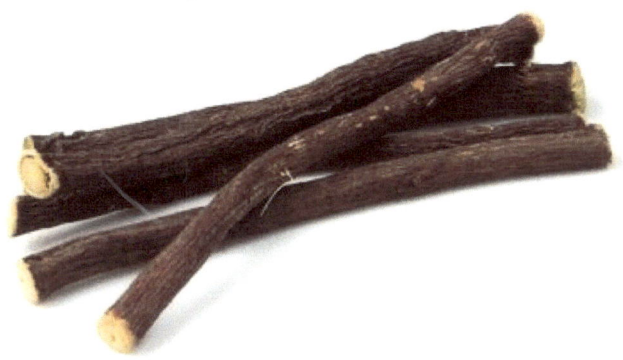

Herbal treatment is now getting appreciation among masses. It's an agreed fact that herbs produce maximum results with minimal side effects. Use of herbs is easy and cost effective as well. Following are the most effective herbal treatments of asthma:

Nettle leaf:

You can use these leaves to make a tea for yourself. You can also mix peppermint and raspberry leaves in this tea. Take these leaves and boil them in few cups of water this it boils. Filter the leaves and add sugar in the tea. Drink this tea 1-2 times each day. This tea is rich in natural anti-histamine substances. Histamine is one of the most potent mediators of inflammation. So, consumption of this tea nullifies the harmful effects of histamine, inhibits its release from mast cells and soothes the air ways.

Peppermint tea:

Peppermint provides a healthy cure for asthma. You can make this tea at home or can use the preparation available in market. For making the tea at home, take peppermint leaves and boil them in water. Filter the water and sugar or honey in it. Drink this tea 1-2 times each day. Peppermint tea helps relieve the symptoms of asthma in following basic ways:

- o It has natural "decongestant" properties. So, it opens up the airway and lessens the symptoms of inflammation seen during asthma.
- o It has a potent anti-histamine effect. It helps suppress the release of histamine and also helps minimize the side effects of histamine.

Eucalyptus oil:

Eucalyptus oil is very effective in curing the problems related to respiratory track. It's particularly effective when used for the treatment of asthma. You can inhale it alone or can add it in boiling water and inhale the steam. It has got potent decongestant properties and helps clear the mucous.

Mustard oil:

A gentle massage of mustard oil is considered an effective herbal remedy for asthma. You can massage you neck, chest and back with this oil. Add 1-2 pinches of camphor in this oil and massage your neck, chest and back with this oil.

Ephedra:

It's a native herbal plant, the leaves of which are used in the treatment of asthma. The leaves of ephedra plant contains a chemical substance known

"Ephedrine". This substance helps relax the spasm of muscles of respiration seen in asthmatic attack. However, this herb is a potent vaso-constrictor and cardio-accelerator and can lead to significant increase in blood pressure. That's why the dosage and frequency of usage should be monitored as per recommendation of an expert.

Coleus Forshkholi:

"Forskolin" is the active ingredient of this herb. This herb decrease the congestion of airway developed during an attack of asthma. However, this herb should not be used by people taking some kind of anti-coagulant drugs because this herb has got a potent anti-coagulant effect of its own and can thus increase the chances of bleeding.

Lobelia:

This herb has got a major effect of curing asthma. Other effects include increasing heart rate and increasing blood pressure.

Reishi mushroom:

This mushroom is very effective herbal remedy for asthma. Its anti-asthmatic activity is attributed to its immune-suppressant activity. It decreases the immune mediated response to irritant and mediators of inflammation. Following are the major functions of this herb:

- o   It suppresses the activity of mast cells, the basic culprit of inflammation and asthma.

- This herb helps relax the muscles of respiratory track and thus helps decrease the congestion and difficulty in breathing caused during asthmatic attack.
- It strengthen lungs, clears the air way and helps in proper respiration.

What to eat, what to avoid?

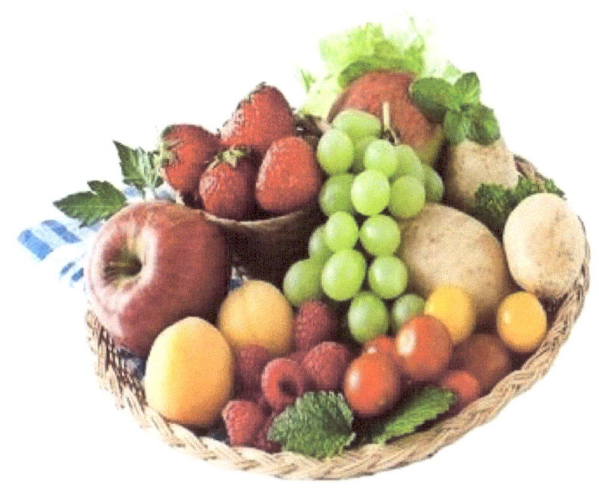

Eating habits matter a lot while treating allergies like asthma because few foods trigger asthma while others help reduce the symptoms. So, having knowledge of the best and the worst food stuff can help you design your eating habits accordingly. It can thus help reduce the intensity as well as the frequency of asthmatic attacks. Following are the eating habits that one should adopt during asthma:

Foods to eat:

Following are the food substances that one should eat during asthma:

- Apples: Apples should be a part of your dining table if you're suffering from asthma. These beneficial effects of apple, in asthma, are attributed to the presence a substance known as "kehllin". Khellin is a natural falvonoid with strong bronco-dilator properties.

- Citrus fruits: Citrus fruits should be used during asthmatic attacks. Citrus fruits are rich source of vitamin C. Vitamin C is a natural anti-oxidant substance which helps decrease the inflammation and constriction of air way produced during asthmatic attack.

- Carrots: Carrots are another food stuff which should be consumed by the patients of asthma. It's rich in beta-carotene, a strong anti-oxidant substance. It helps stabilize the membranes of mast cells and help suppress the adverse effects of inflammation.

- Garlic: Garlic is used for the treatment of several health related conditions, asthma is one of such conditions. It decreases the blockade of airway caused during asthma. You can use garlic in several ways:
  - Take almost 10-15 cloves of garlic and add them in a cup of milk. Heat the milk till it becomes Luke warm. Cool the milk and drink it once daily.
  - Or you can add 3-4 cloves of garlic in a cup of water and heat it till it becomes Luke water. Filter the water and drink it 1-2 times each day.
  - You can simply increase the use of garlic in your meals, salads and soups.

- Ginger: Ginger is an effective treatment for several health related conditions. You can use ginger in several ways:
  - You can simply add it in your daily meals, soups, drinks or salads.
  - You can make a tea with garlic. Take small amount of garlic and heat it after adding it into 1-2 cups of water. Heat this water

till it boils. Cool it and filter the ginger out. You can consume this tea 1-2 times each day.

o Take 2 table spoons of soaked and grinded fenugreek seeds, 1 tea spoon of honey and 1 tea spoon of garlic powder and mix all these components. Use this mixture once in the morning for maximum results.

- Salmon fish: Salmon fish is rich in omega-3 fatty acid. Omega-3 fatty acid is a natural anti-oxidant substance. It decreases the inflammation and helps abate the symptoms of inflammation.

- Figs: Eating figs also helps reduce the symptoms of asthma. It helps improve the respiration and help the expulsion of phlegm.

- Onions: Onions are also very effective for the patients of asthma. You can use onions in your meals or can eat them raw in salads.

- Flaxseeds: Flaxseeds, whole, grinded, soaked or dried, can be used in intense asthmatic attacks. It's a rich source of omega-3 fatty acid. Omega-3 fatty acid helps reduce inflammation and all the side effects associated with it.

  Flaxseeds are also a rich source of magnesium. Magnesium is responsible for causing the relaxation of muscles of respiration. So, asthmatic patients should make flaxseeds a part of their regular diet.

- Milk: Milk is also very effective in curing asthma. It contains a high amount of vitamin D. Vitamin D is a potent anti-oxidant and has got valuable role in suppressing inflammation.

- Avocado: Avocado contains an important anti-oxidant substance known as "glutathione". The presence of this anti-oxidant makes avocado the best food stuff for asthma.

- Water: Keeping yourself hydrated can help fight the symptoms of asthma. So, drink at least 8-10 glasses of water each day.

Foods to avoid:

There are certain food substances that act as trigger for the release of chemical mediators of inflammation. So, such food substances should be avoided during asthma. Such food includes:

- Egg: Egg should be avoided in all types of immune reactions, especially asthma. Eating eggs can trigger intense reaction which can sometimes produce deleterious side effects.

- Dairy products: Milk is effective in the treatment of asthma. But, the use of dairy products, like cheese, should be strictly avoided during asthma. Some people show intense reaction to the consumption of such dairy products.

- Spices: If you're suffering from asthma then you've to be careful about the level of spices in your daily meals. You might like spicy food but using a spice free food is a pre-requisite in the treatment of asthma.

- Peanuts: Peanuts are the worst nightmare for the patients of asthma. A single nut can trigger intense obstruction and can, thus, produce fatal results. So, the use of peanut and peanut containing products should be strictly avoided by the patients of asthma.

- Shellfish: Trout and salmon fish are rich in omega-3 fatty acid and should be used by the patients of asthma. However, shellfish is the worst thing to eat if you're a patient of asthma. Shellfish allergy is the third leading food allergy.

- Wine: Most of the wines contain sulfites as the preservatives. So, the use of wine should be avoided during asthma.
  However, some studies suggest that wine contains a natural substance called "libation". This compound can actually decrease the symptoms of asthma. So, small quantity of wine can actually help in abating the symptoms of asthma.

Healthy life style – An effective prophylaxis

Sometimes, simple life style changes can bring major effects on your life. In most of the cases, an unhealthy life style and poor hygiene trigger intense asthmatic attacks. In such conditions, adopting a healthy style can prove to be extremely beneficial in the treatment of asthma. This may sound insignificant, but such changes can significantly decrease the frequency of asthmatic attack and can act as an effective prophylaxis. Life style changes in asthma include:

- **Use air conditioners:**
  Use your air conditioners to keep the air around you clean and free of pollutant. Air conditioners help reduce the chance of development of asthma due to following basic reasons:
  - Air conditioners have got air cleaning systems in them. They clean the air of all the smoke, dust and pollen particles. So, they make the air clean and safe to breathe.
  - Air conditioners help keep the level of humidity inside a room within an optimum level. Too much or too low humidity can trigger asthmatic attack. So, air conditioners help keep asthma away by checking the room level of humidity.

  It's best to keep your room door closed during the seasons of pollen and allergy.

- **Clean your room décor:**
  Most of the people don't have any idea that the basic trigger of asthma lies right next to them. Untidy pillows, mattresses and box springs provide an excellent habitat for mites and cockroaches to

breed. Moreover, with time the quantity of dust increases in this room stuff. So, it's advised to clean your pillows and bed sheets regularly. Moreover, you should replace the carpets with wooden or linoleum floors so that the floor doesn't get contaminated with dust and other irritants.

- **Reduce mould spore:**
Mould spores are present everywhere in the atmosphere. Cold and dark places provide an excellent habitat for the mould to grow and produce spores. Look around you and you'll see that your house is full of such areas. Mould usually grows in washrooms, wash basins, damp floors and clothes. So, you should be extra careful and clean all such areas. This way, you can limit the production of mould spores and attacks of asthma.

- **Reduce pet dander:**
Sometimes, the basic source of allergy is nothing else but your beloved pets. Pets hoard several triggers for asthma, like:
  - The hair shedding from the body may trigger an intense asthmatic response in an individual.
  - The excreta of pets, when inhaled or accidently ingested, may serve as a trigger for asthma.
  - The wastes of pets sometimes contain several worm or other micro-organisms, which when gain entry to the human body, can start an intense asthmatic attack.
  - The hair of cats and dogs harbor several insects, like mites. These insects are the basic culprit of asthma in sensitive individuals.

So, you should be vigilant enough while having a pet in your house. You should follow some guideline regarding the cleanliness of your house and pet.

- o Always keep your pet clean. Give it proper bath on regular intervals.
- o Get it checked from a doctor if it shows some signs of infection or disease.
- o Make sure your house remains clean of the wastes of your pet.
- o If you are an asthmatic then it's best not to handle the pets altogether.
- o Wear mask and procure extra protection while cleaning your pet.

- **Cover your mouth and nose:**
  It may sound very simple and one may get skeptic about the effectiveness of this method. But, the truth is, it's the most effective prophylactic measure for asthma. The basic reason being that most of the allergens and pollutants get entry into the respiratory track through nose or mouth. You should wear a mask:
  - o When you go outside as it would save you from dust, smoke and chemical.
  - o When you are driving your car, bike or bicycle as it would save it from the fumes of burning fuel.
  - o When you go outside during the season of pollens.
  - o When you're handling your pets.

- **Stay healthy:**

  Adopting a healthy life style is one of the basic pre-requisite for the treatment of asthma. Following are some points which are note worthy:

  - **Get regular exercise:** If you're suffering from asthma then it doesn't mean that you've to sit inside your room all the times. A regular exercise is very important in preventing asthma. Getting a regular exercise doesn't mean that you've to be a marathon runner. A regular exercise for 20-30 minutes each day should do the trick. You can start with simple exercises like brisk walking, jogging or running. Regular exercise helps strengthen your heart and helps improve the health of your lungs.

  - **Maintain a normal weight:** Obesity is one of the most important risk factors for asthma. So, you should try to lose your weight. Eat healthy, get regular exercise and don't get stressed. Losing extra weight should help a lot in reducing the risk of asthma.

  - **Eat healthy:** As described earlier, eat a lot of fruits and vegetables rich in anti-oxidant, minerals and omega-3 fatty acids. But every vegetables and fruit is not suitable, as some fruits and vegetables can trigger an asthmatic attack.

  - **Control heart burn:** The reflux of acid from the stomach can cause the erosion of respiratory track and can thus increase the chances of development of asthma. So, you should try to avoid heart burn as much as possible.

Photo credits

All images licensed by fotolia.com

Obst und Gemüse

© *PhotoSG - Fotolia.com*

Washing Hands

© *MaksimKostenko - Fotolia.com*

bastoncini di liquirizia

© *Lsantilli - Fotolia.com*

asthma inhaler

© *Jenny Thompson - Fotolia.com*

Husten

© *Klaus Eppele - Fotolia.com*

Allergies

© *kbuntu - Fotolia.com*

Kaffce

© *jogyx - Fotolia.com*

inhalation

© *photomim - Fotolia.com*

female surgeon with surgical team

© *beerkoff - Fotolia.com.*

Author Bio

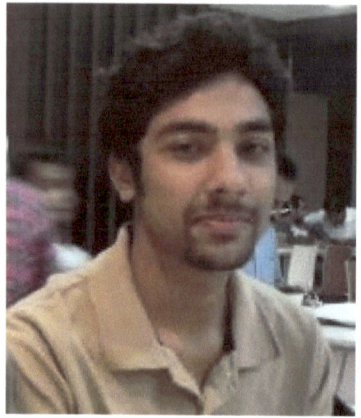

Muhammad Usman is a distinguished medical graduate of Allama iqbal medical college (AIMC). He is a professional writer who has been in the field for more than 4 years. During this time he has produced 10,000+ articles, blogs and eBooks on various niches related to diseases, health, fitness, nutrition and well-being. He is a regular contributor to several journals related to medicine and surgery. He is the editor of several journals and newspapers.

Check out some of the other JD-Biz Publishing books

Gardening Series on Amazon

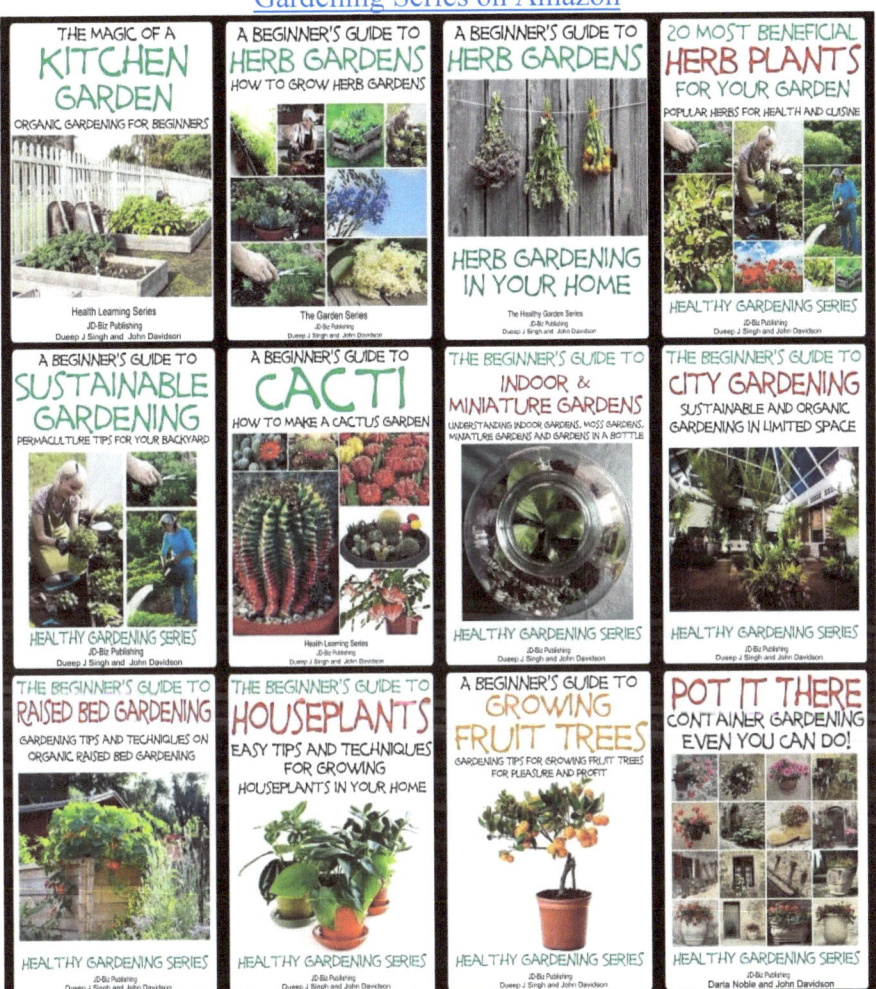

Health Learning Series

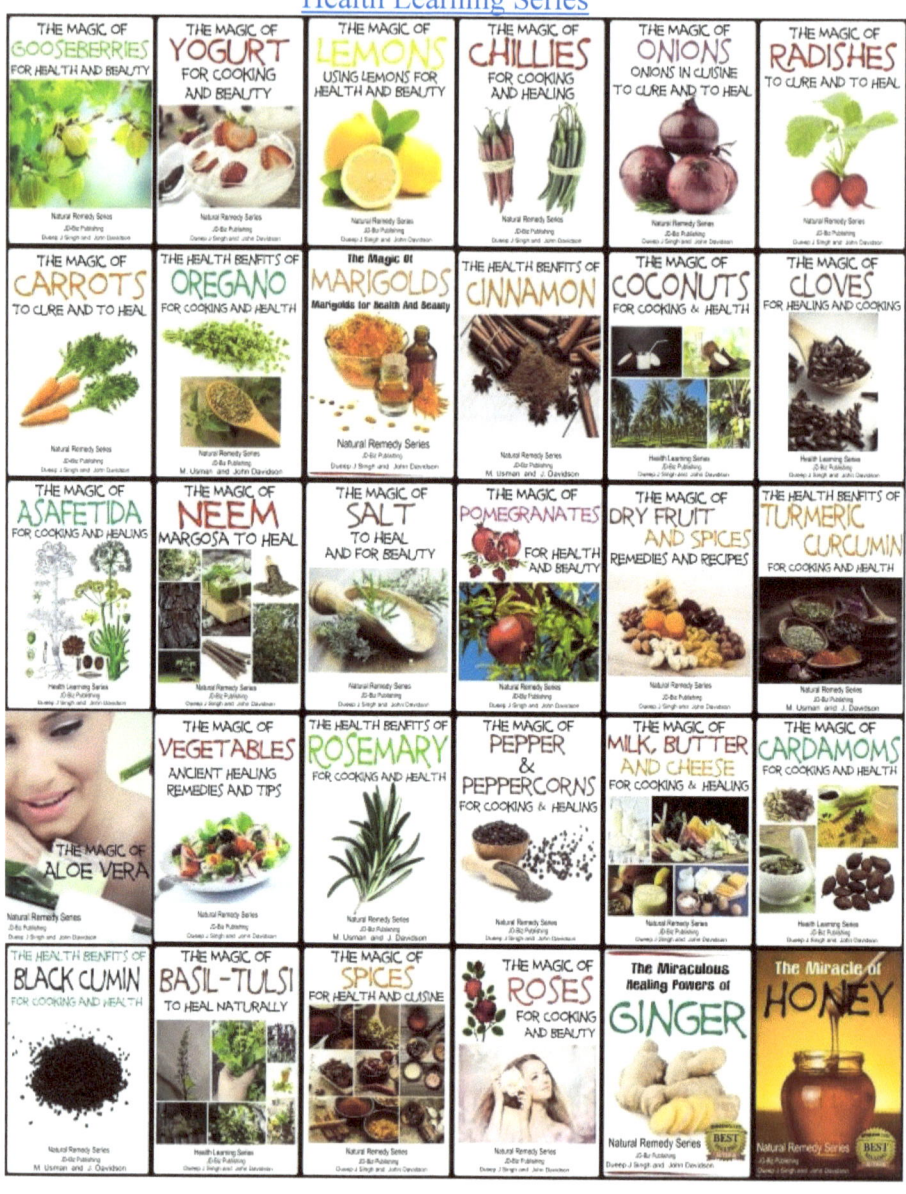

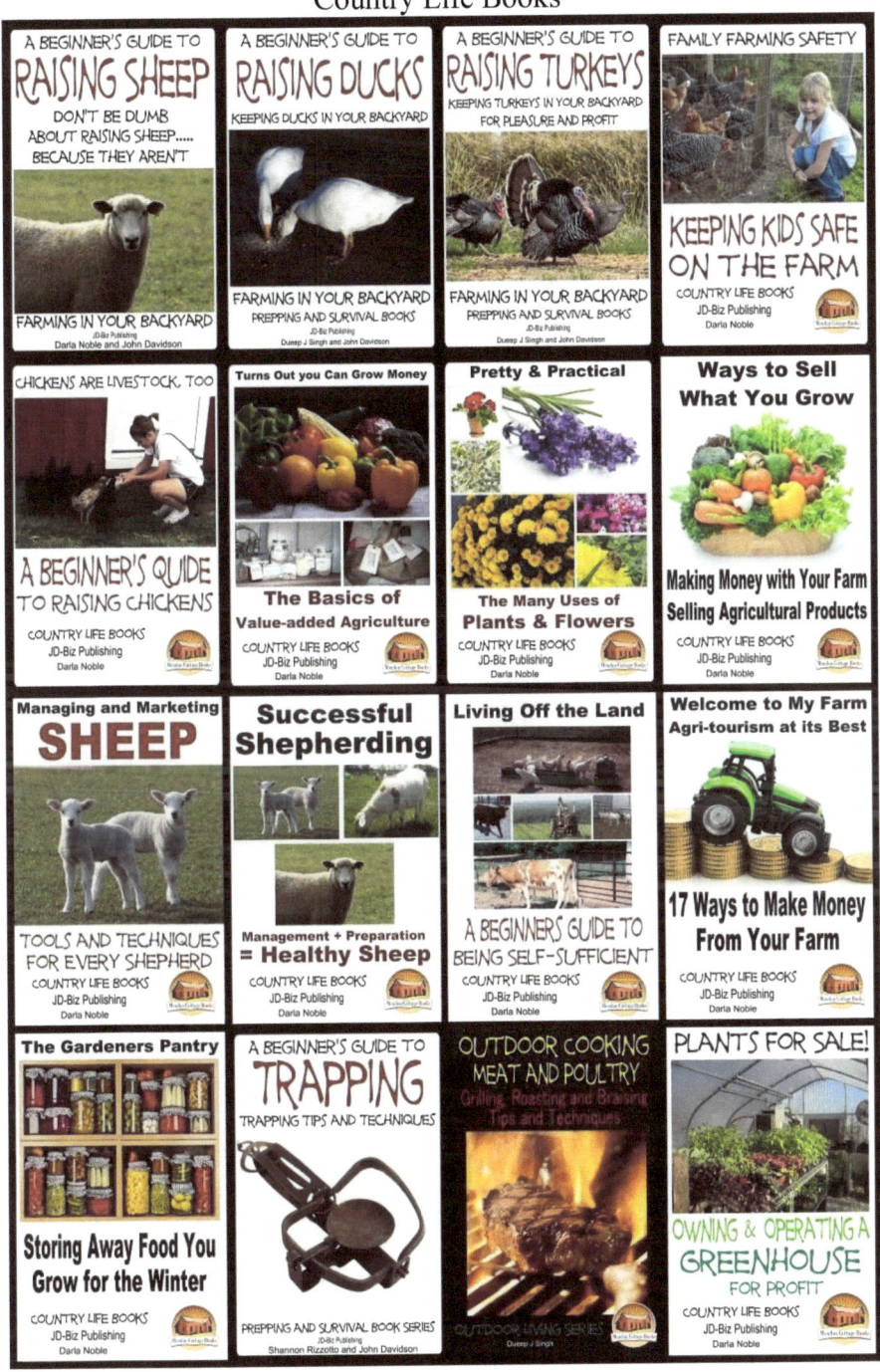

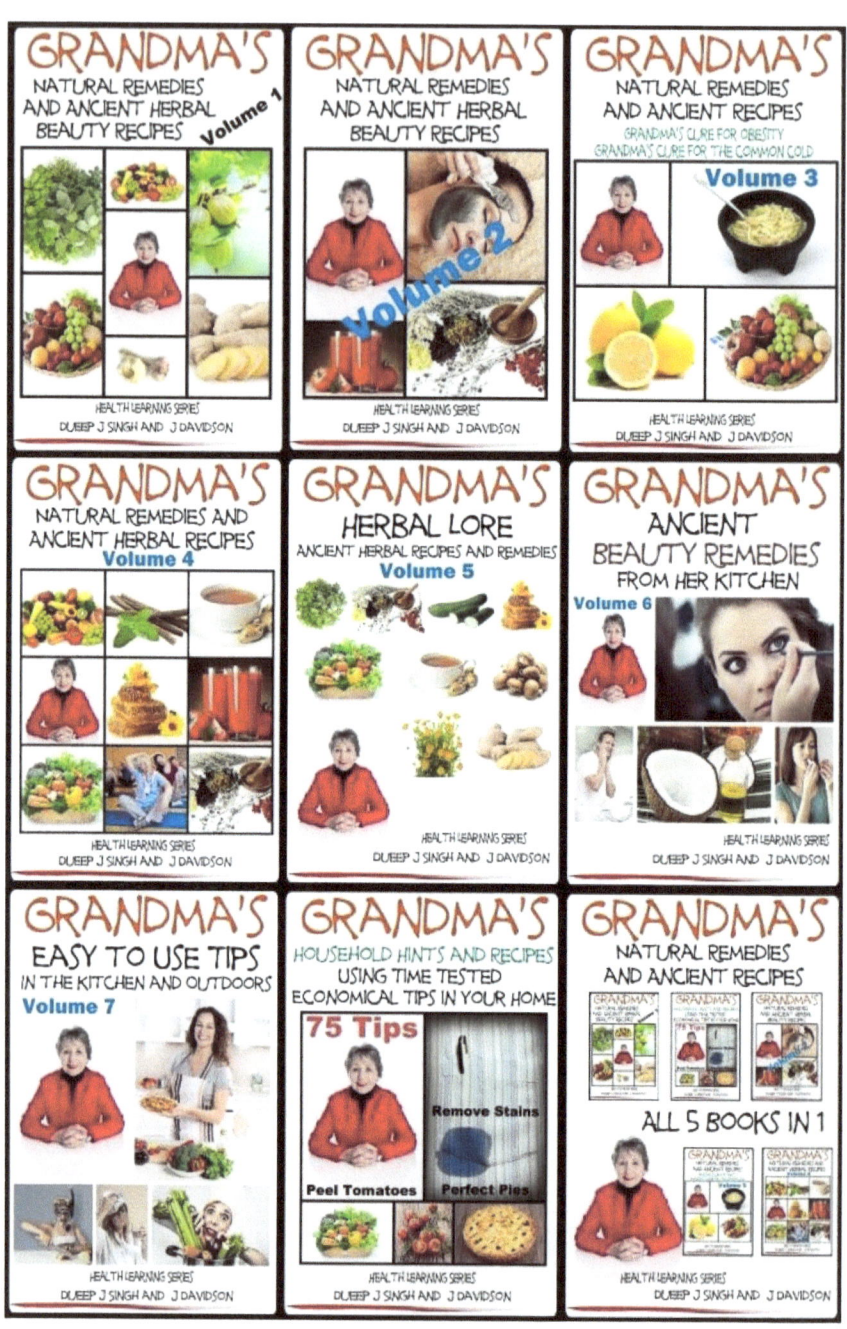

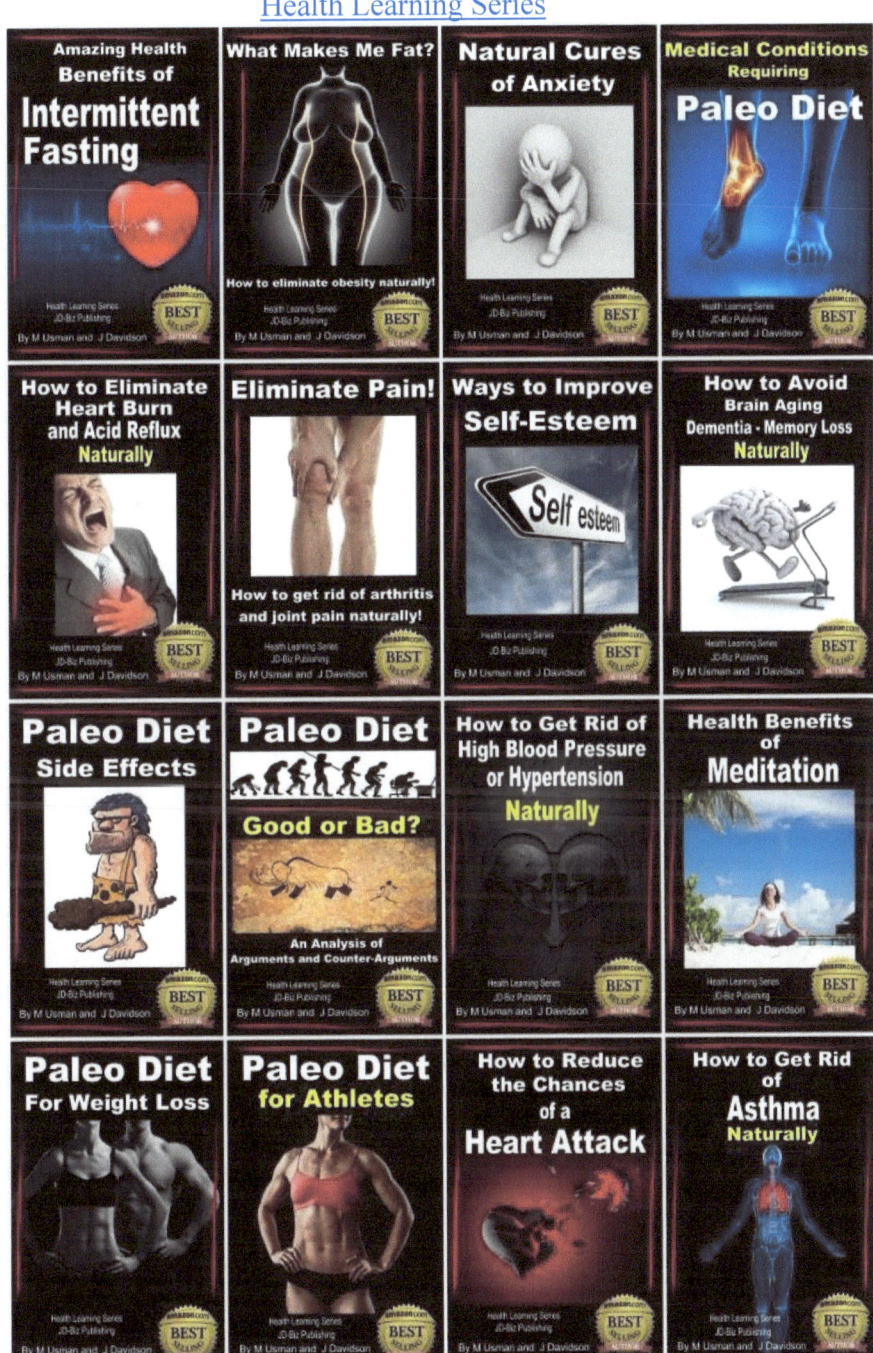

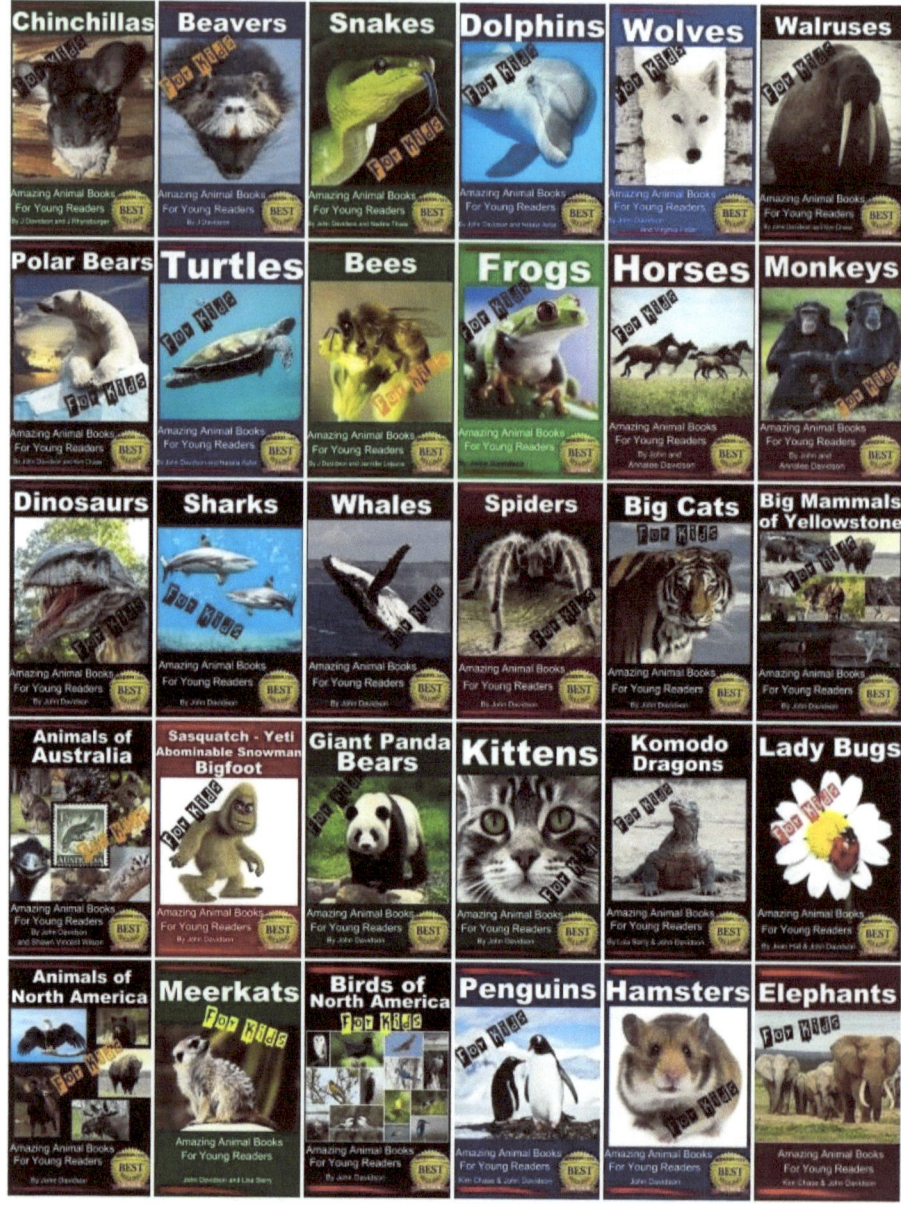

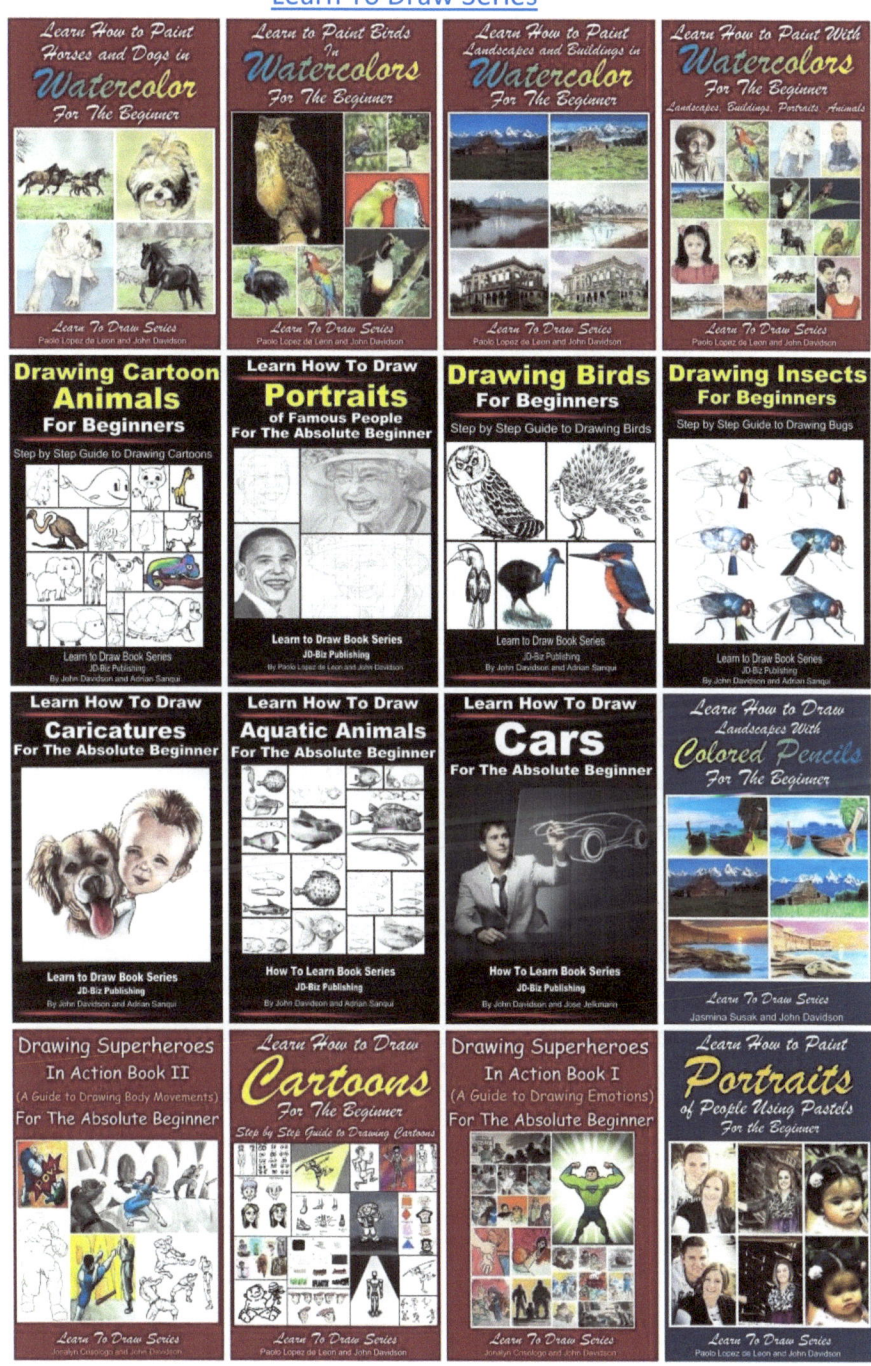

How to Build and Plan Books

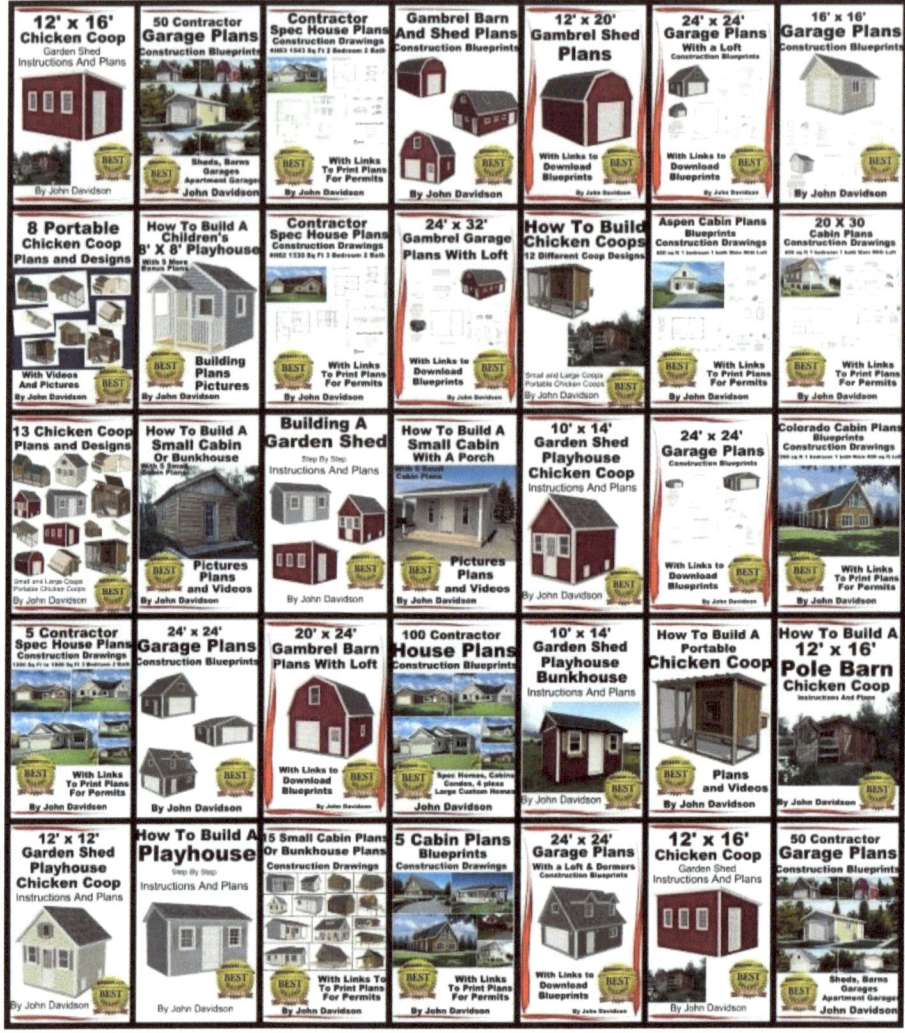

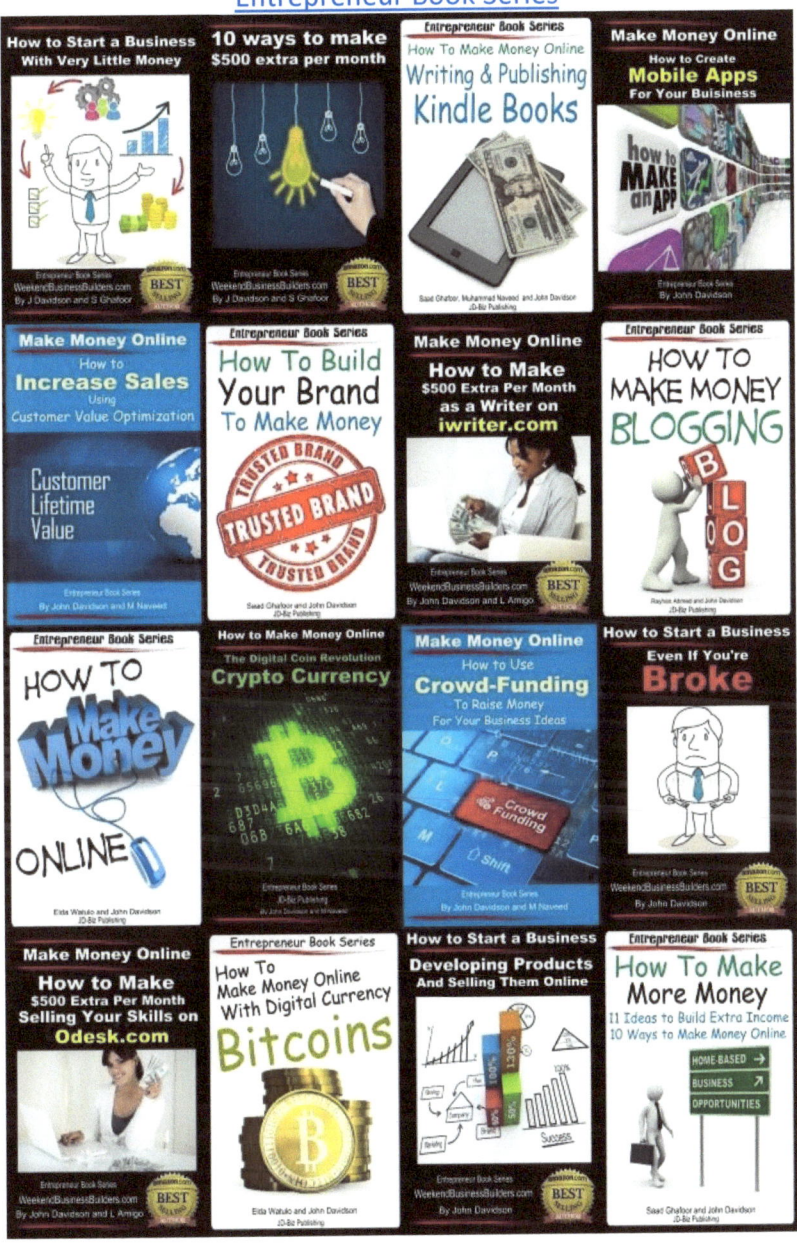

Our books are available at

1. Amazon.com
2. Barnes and Noble
3. Itunes
4. Kobo
5. Smashwords
6. Google Play Books

Download Free Books!
http://MendonCottageBooks.com

Publisher

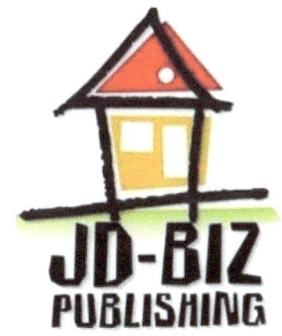

JD-Biz Corp

P O Box 374

Mendon, Utah 84325

http://www.jd-biz.com/

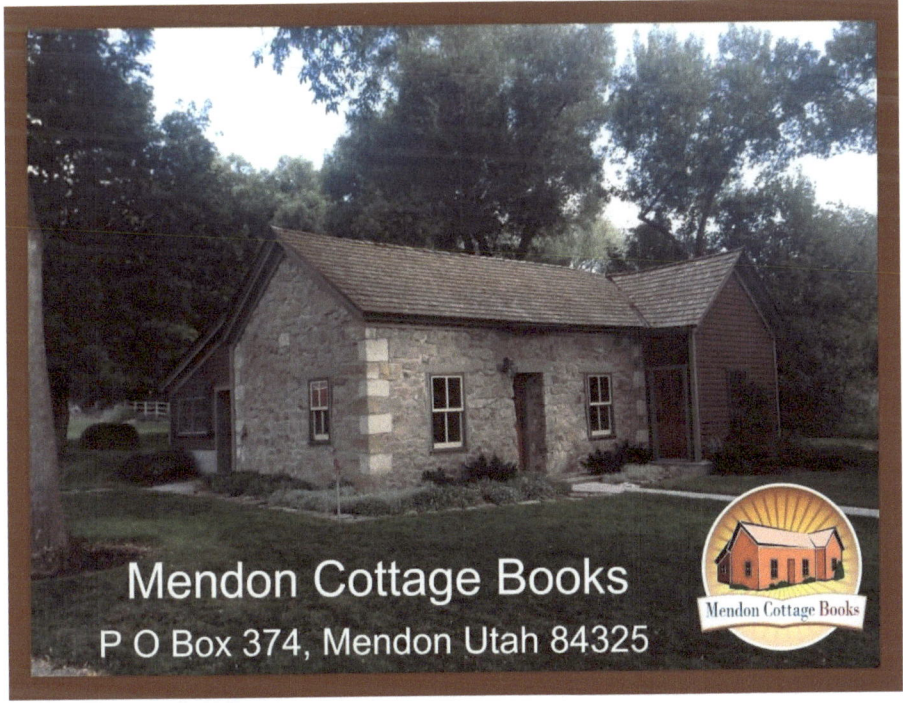

Mendon Cottage Books

P O Box 374, Mendon Utah 84325

www.ingramcontent.com/pod-product-compliance
Lightning Source LLC
Chambersburg PA
CBHW050840290526
45792CB00001B/479

Desert Tortoise

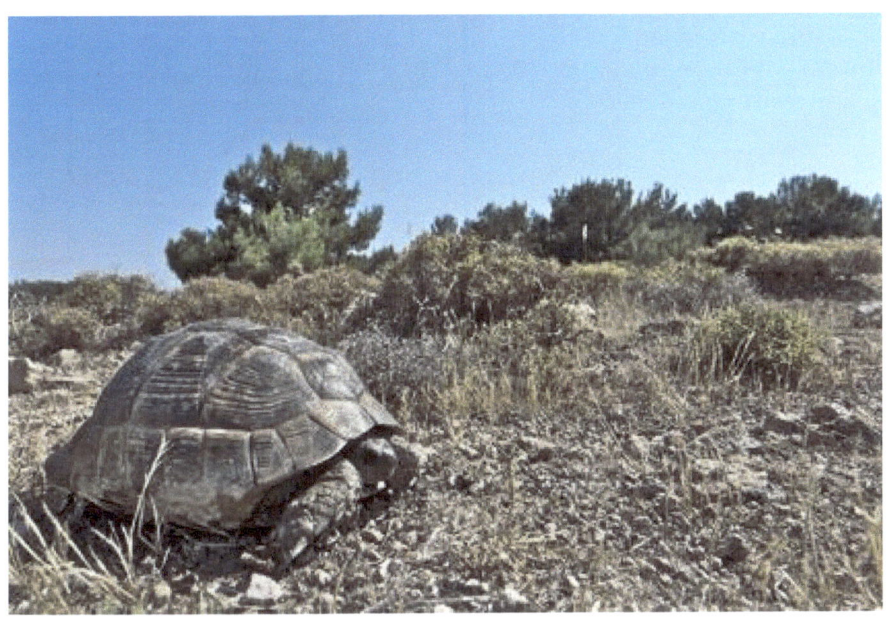

The desert tortoise is a type of tortoise which is medium in size. The size of it can vary from 9 to 15 inches usually. These tortoises can live up-to 80 years and they are known for their long lifetime.

Desert tortoises require the suitable environment to live. So if anyone wants to pet them he should provide the necessary things like a large aquarium and proper food. The aquarium floor should be covered with papers, garden dirt or pallets of rabbit.

Most of the people don't know that these creatures are highly sensitive to excessive humidity. Hay protect them as hay can hold excessive humidity. Now you know this fact which most of the people don't know.

These tortoises like to eat grasses, shrubs, new grown cacti and their flowers. But if there is a shortage of food they can manage to dry forage too

Sea Tortoise

We have come to the sea turtle section. You will be fascinated to learn that sea turtles come in various sizes and attractive colors. As they have cold blood, they are categorized in the reptile species. Which means that they are partly related to lizard, crocodiles or snakes.

These seas are found all over the world. Some of them prefers to live in the tropical waters and others like the places where water is cooler. They roam around the open sea in search of food. Sea turtles are widely known as one of the most ancient creatures. They are on earth about 110 million. In that time dinosaurs also existed.

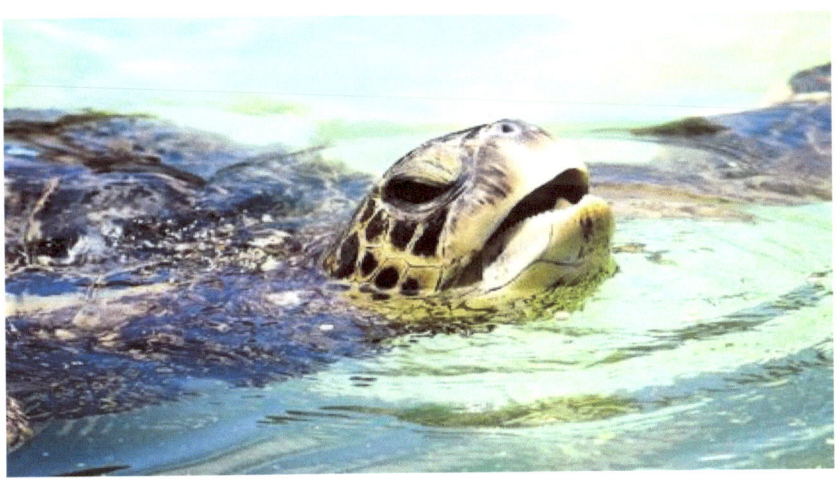

Sea turtles are a bit different from other turtles as they cannot retract their legs and head into their shells. Seven types of sea turtles are found nowadays. Green sea turtle, leatherback sea turtle , Flatback sea turtle is amongst those types. These names depend on their colors. Sea turtles depend on sea animals and plants for their living and they spend more time under water.

Giant Tortoise

Galapagos tortoise is renowned by the name giant tortoise. There is a reason behind calling it a giant tortoise and that is because it is the world's largest tortoise. As it is large it is also the earth's heaviest tortoise. Each one can weight up-to 900 pounds and the length of its shell can be up-to 54 inches.

These types of tortoises require huge ground for grazing and they usually live on tropical islands. Keeping a giant tortoise as a pet is almost impossible mostly because of its size and habits. They can't be kept indoors.

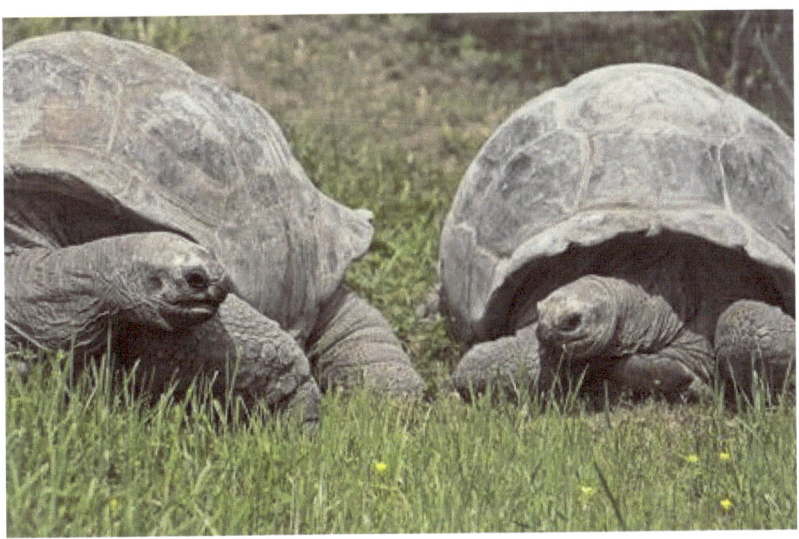

What do they eat? This is a common question to all. The good news is that they are vegetarians. They eat grasses, leaves, fruits, cactus in large quantity. For this reason they are also referred as eating machines. Well the amazing fact is that they can store food and water for a long time.

Unfortunately for us, these giant tortoises are facing extinction problem. A few of their species are surviving. A few people killed them for their petty selfishness. Thousands of these tortoises were killed for their skin, shell and oil. Though the remaining of them are being protected by the law, many people are still killing them. Now, zoo is the only place where we can find them.

Green Turtle

The green turtle is a kind of sea turtle which is also known as pacific green turtle or black turtle. These turtles are mostly largest amongst marine turtles. And they are the only plant eaters among other sea turtles. The adult ones depend mostly on shallow lagoons.

Green turtles have flattened body which is covered by the carapace. This carapace is smooth and mainly light colored although eastern pacific ones are black.

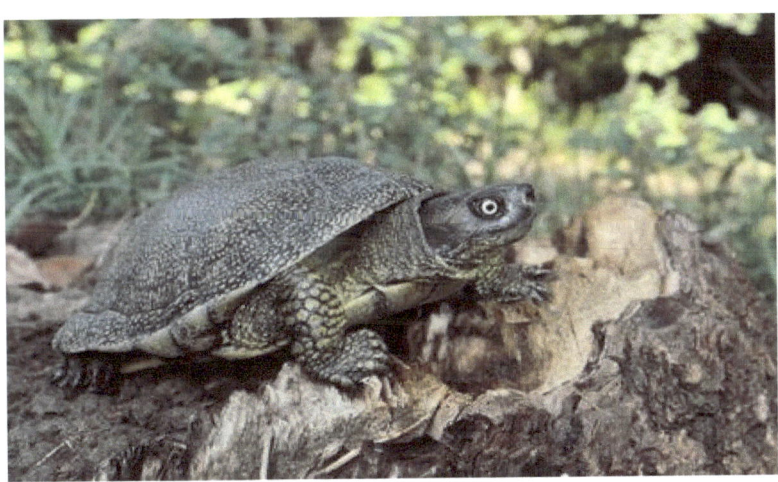

They are like other marine turtles who migrate long distances for laying their eggs. Green turtles are endangered species who are going to extinct soon if serious steps are not taken. They are threatened by the fishers and people around their egg laying site.

Do you know an interesting fact about them? They help to make the sea grass and algae more productive by grazing.

Box Turtle

When we hear the word box what usually comes to our mind? Obviously the shape of it or image of it floats in our mind. The same we can say about box turtle or tortoise because it is shaped like a box.

These turtles are mainly from North America and they are terrestrial. But they spend a little bit of time in the shallow water.

Anyone can keep box turtle as a pet because they are very lovely creatures. But that person has to think twice. Are you thinking why? That's because because most turtle experts say to keep the box turtles outdoors and not everybody can do so.

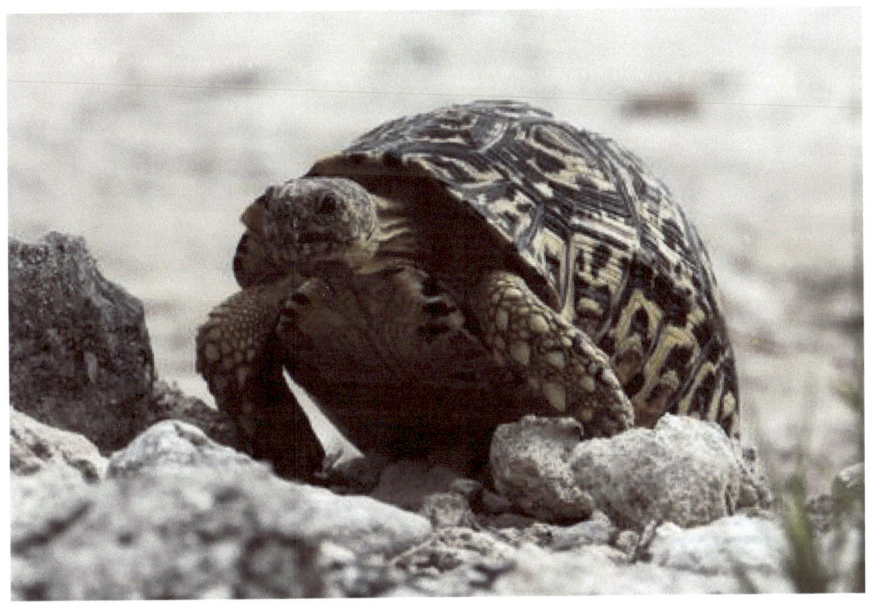

The box turtles have several species but most of them look alike. So we have to differentiate them by some other ways.

What does this turtle eat?

Well, like most turtles they are omnivores but basically they eat what they get. When they are between 5-6 years they are mainly carnivorous.

Loggerhead Turtle

Loggerhead is a type of sea turtle which is distributed around the world. These turtles can grow up-to 279 cm. But usually up to 90cm when fully grown and weighs 300 pounds. Their skin has a color range from yellow to brown and their shell's color is usually reddish brown.

They cannot be easily hunted compared to other turtles. Loggerhead turtle has powerful jaws which is supported by their large heads and this is also the reason behind calling it by this name.

Loggerhead sea turtles are mainly seen around the Atlantic, Pacific or Indian Oceans. They spend their lifetime under saltwater but females come to lay their eggs at the shores. They feed mainly on invertebrates.

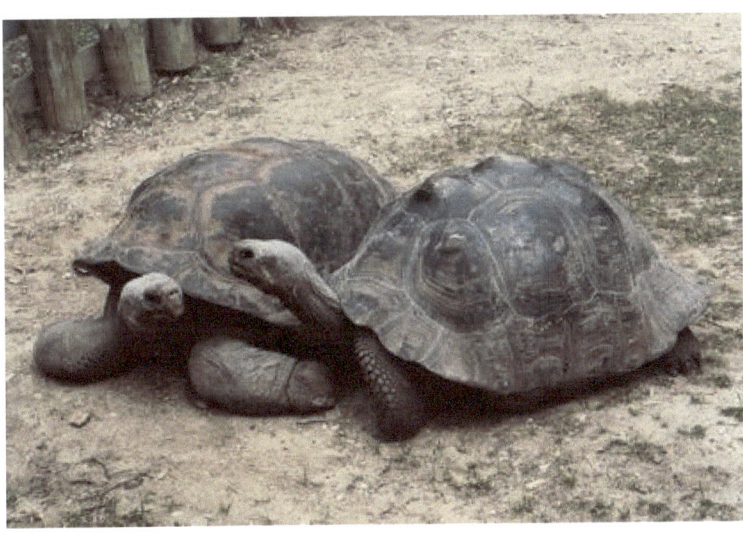

These sea turtles move slowly and defenselessly on the land though they are swift in the ocean. As only female come to lay eggs on land they do this job carefully so nothing can harm their eggs.

Interesting Facts About the Tortoise

Who doesn't like to know interesting or exciting things? So here are some facts about tortoises which will amaze everyone.

- The evolution of tortoises happened before the mammals, lizards, snakes. Tortoises are one of the ancient creatures living on earth.

- 60 different bones make tortoise's shell which are connected to each other.

- Most of the tortoise can live a long life like a hundred years of age.

- Most living animals have teeth but tortoises don't have them.

- The tortoise has a bony portion in its shell which protects it from many dangers.

- The desert tortoise can survive ground temperature exceeding 140 degree Fahrenheit.

- Tortoises who are adult can survive many years without water

- Most of the land tortoises have carapaces which are high doomed. This protects them from the jaws of terrestrial predators.

- They have an extreme smell sense and a good eyesight.

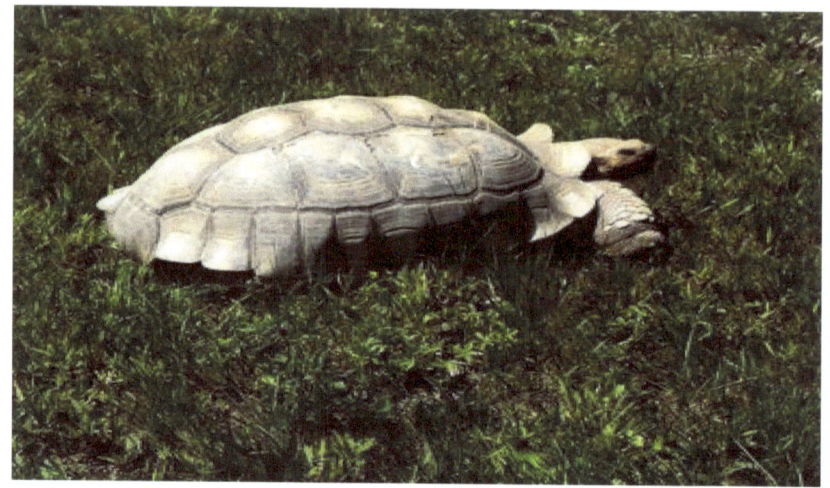

- They have a long life because of their shells which are both strong and unique.

- Most female tortoises lay 2-12 eggs and they put their eggs in deep holes to save the eggs from predators. The eggs hatch in around 90-120 days.

- Most male tortoises have longer tails than female ones.

- Tortoises don't have flippers but turtles do.

There are many interesting tortoise facts which are still left untold. If you wish to have tortoise as a pet then you should keep these facts in your mind. These facts will help you in understanding your pet tortoise properly.

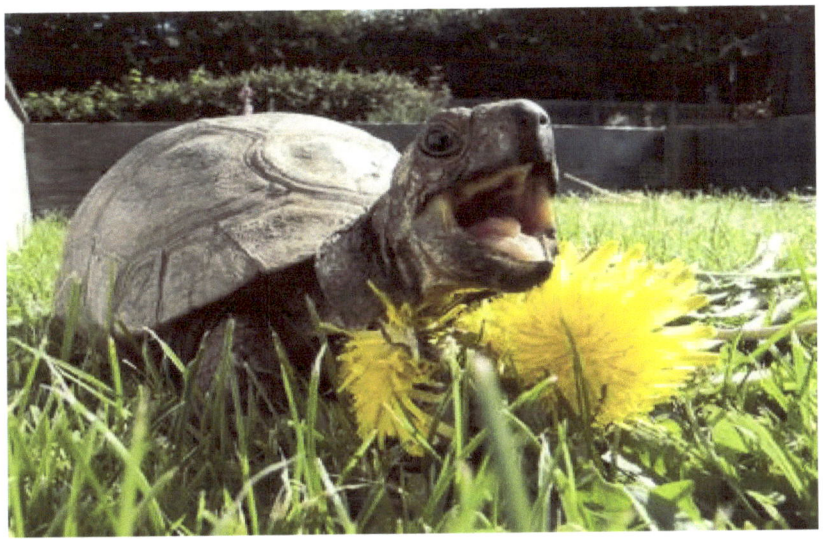

Turtle Facts

Facts are a kind of statement which are true and sometimes it is contrasted with opinion and beliefs. Facts usually fascinate every age of people from kids to adults. Humans still don't know any facts about turtles which are necessary to know. Here some facts based on turtle are given below:

- If someone thinks that his pet turtle will become very old after a few years, he is definitely wrong. Because most turtles become juvenile at the age of 80.

- If someone's pet turtle lays eggs then he will have to wait for at least two months as the eggs need incubation.

- It is a common fact that turtles are slow but people don't know that green sea turtles can run 20 miles per hour when they are being attacked by someone or feel endangered by something. Turtles can see an extra color which humans cannot see.

- Scientists call turtle's shell "dust bag".

- Some turtles have a temperament which is very snappy. In this case it can cause damage like biting someone for the silliest causes. If anyone has this sort of turtle he should be aware of it and observe the temperament.

- Most of the sea turtles can swim swiftly. This speed can go up-to 35 miles per hour depending on the turtle type and situation. They are really fast, aren't they?

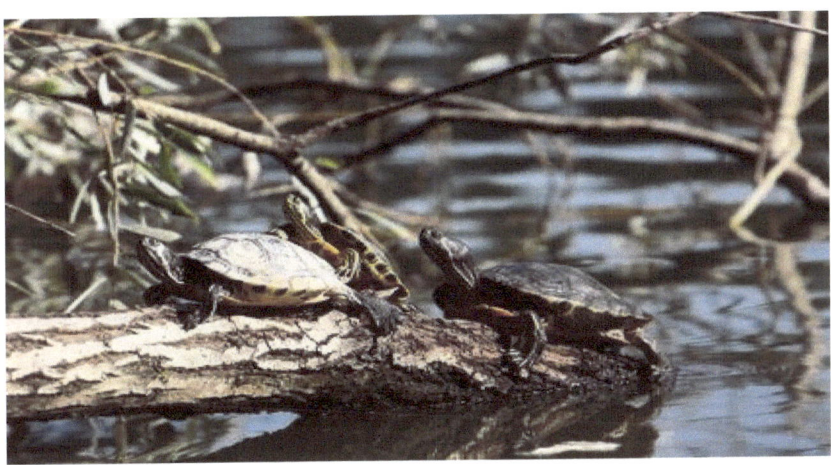

- Some people believe that sea turtles cry if they are unhappy. But the scientific fact is that they just excrete salt which is excess, through the medium of tears. So, if you own a sea turtle now do not get the wrong idea that your turtle is sad.

- Do you know what the baby turtles are called? They are called sparkies. Isn't it interesting?

Read More Amazing Animal Books

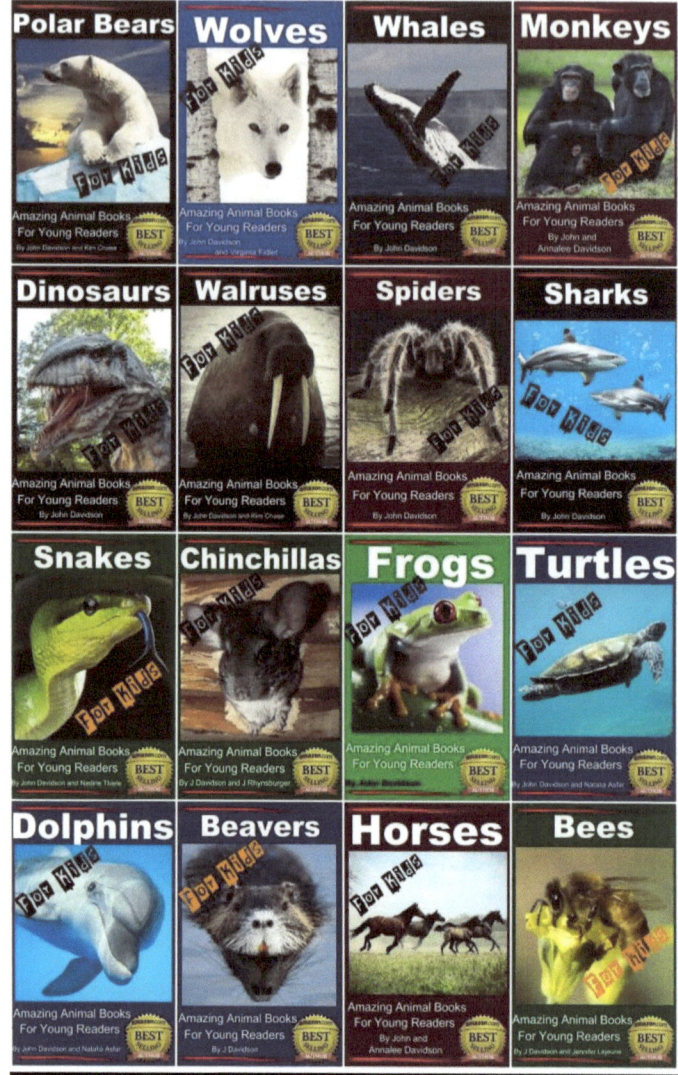

Purchase at Amazon.com
Website http://AmazingAnimalBooks.com

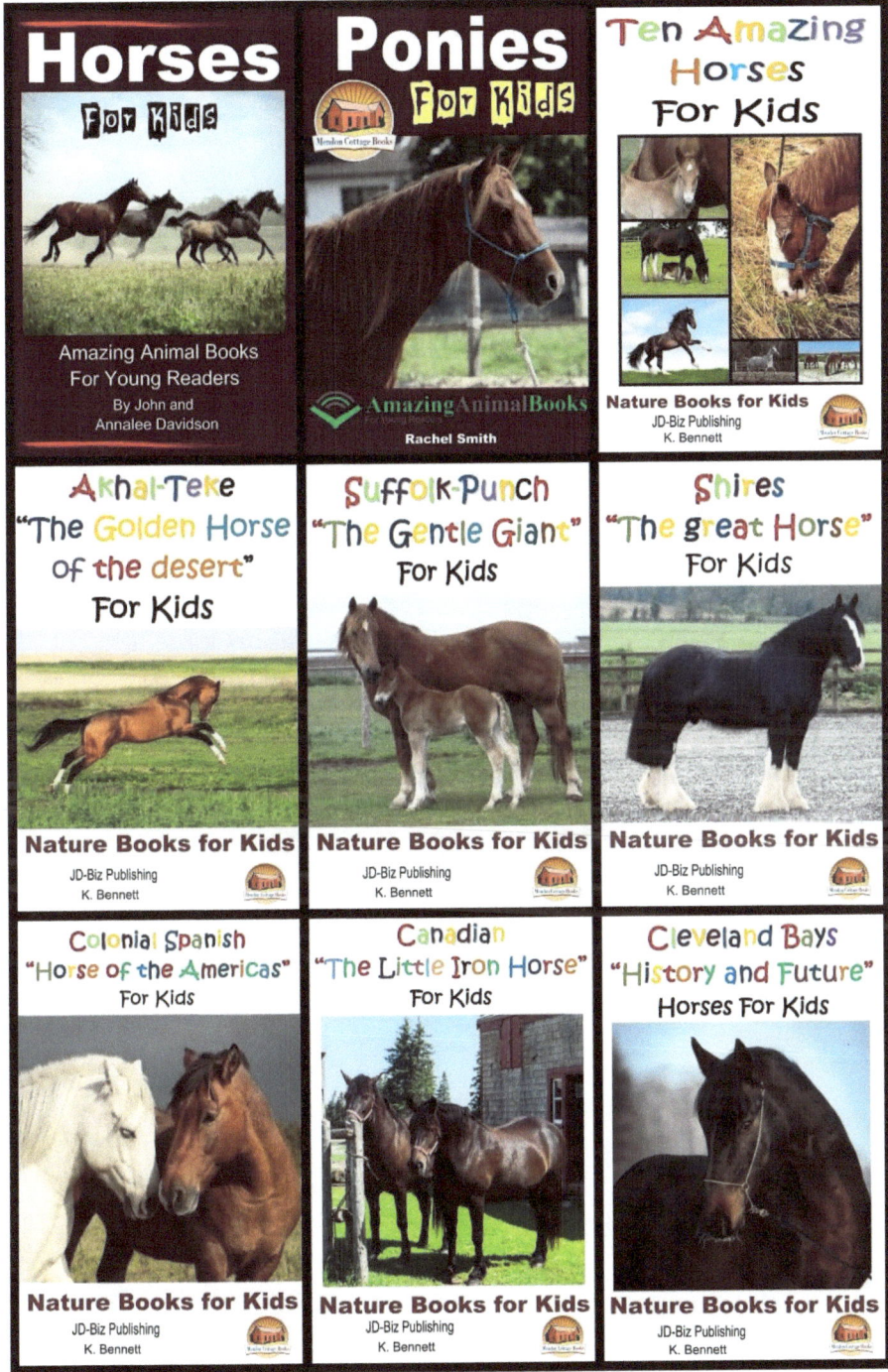

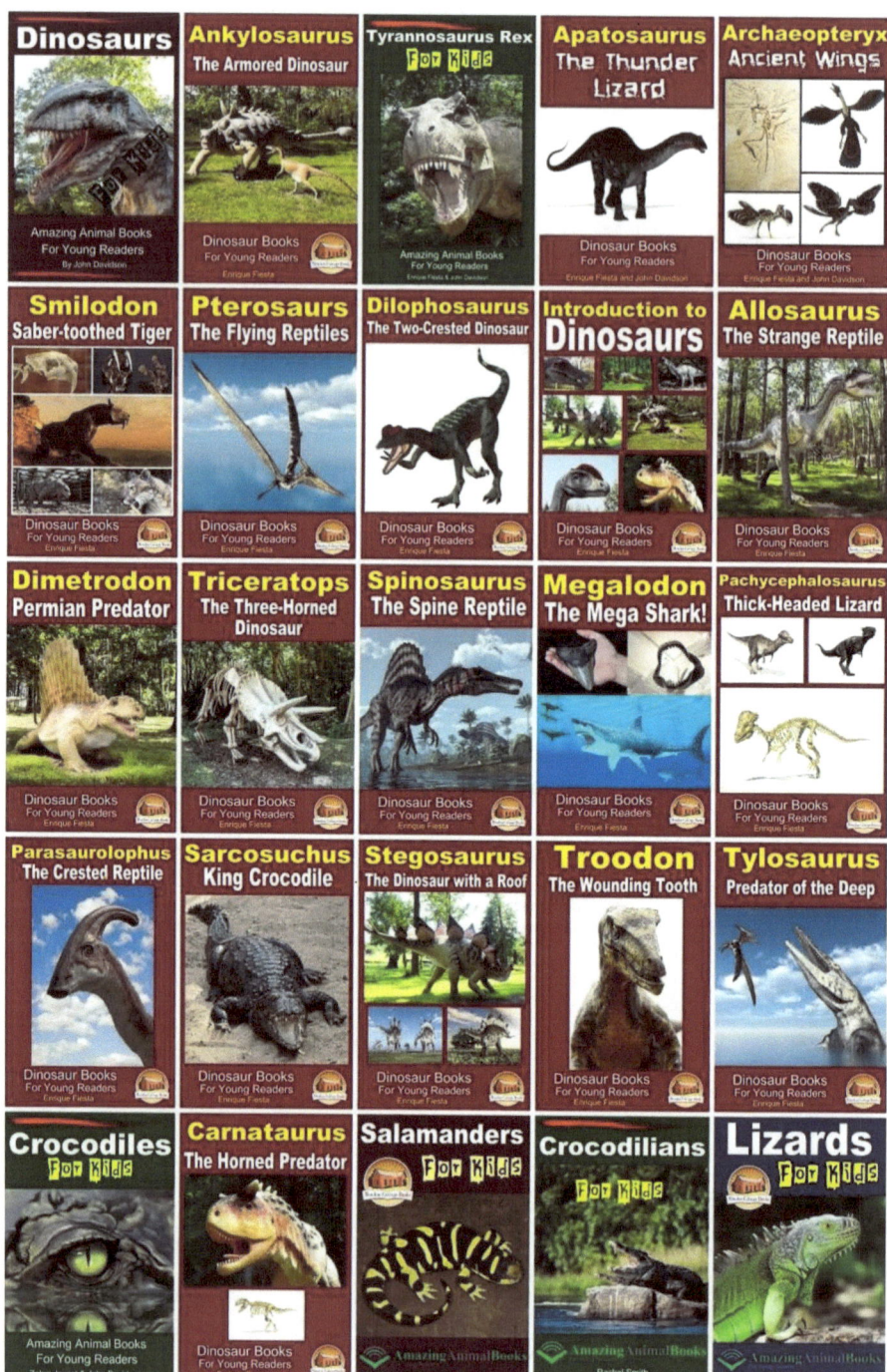

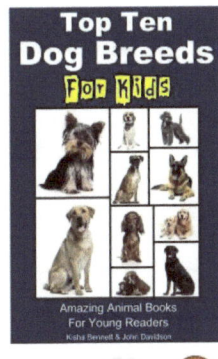

Top Ten Dog Breeds For Kids
Amazing Animal Books For Young Readers
Kisha Bennett & John Davidson

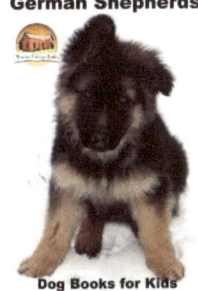

German Shepherds
Dog Books for Kids
K. Bennett

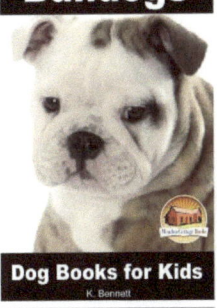

Bulldogs
Dog Books for Kids
K. Bennett

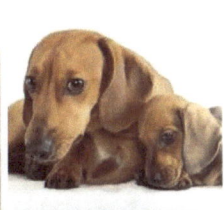

Dachshund
Dog Books for Kids
K. Bennett

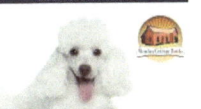

Poodles
Dog Books for Kids
K. Bennett

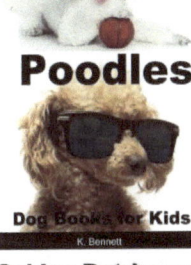

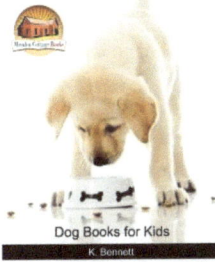

Labrador Retrievers
Dog Books for Kids
K. Bennett

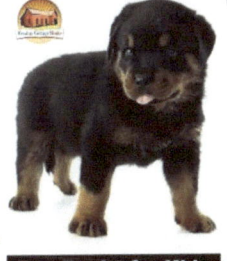

Rottweilers
Dog Books for Kids
K. Bennett

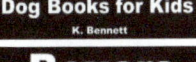 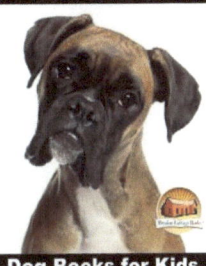

Boxers
Dog Books for Kids
K. Bennett

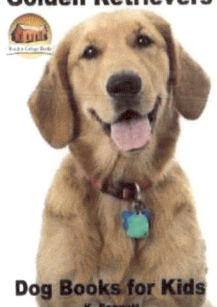

Golden Retrievers
Dog Books for Kids
K. Bennett

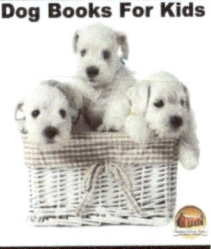

Puppies
Dog Books For Kids
Amazing Animal Books
By John Davidson

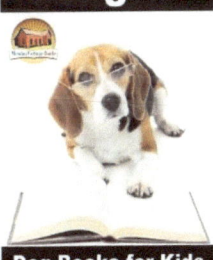

Beagles
Dog Books for Kids
K. Bennett

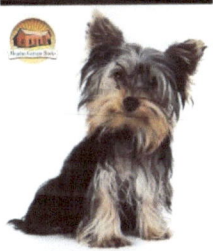

Yorkshire Terriers
Dog Books for Kids
K. Bennett

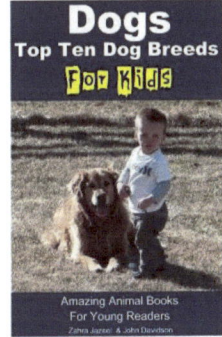

Dogs
Top Ten Dog Breeds For Kids
Amazing Animal Books For Young Readers
Zahra Jazeel & John Davidson

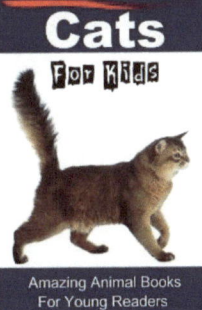

Cats For Kids
Amazing Animal Books For Young Readers
K. Bennett & John Davidson

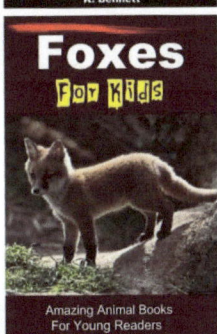 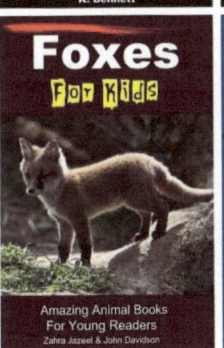

Foxes For Kids
Amazing Animal Books For Young Readers
Zahra Jazeel & John Davidson

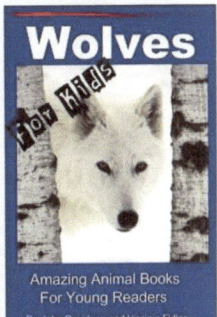

Wolves For Kids
Amazing Animal Books For Young Readers
By John Davidson and Virginia Fidler

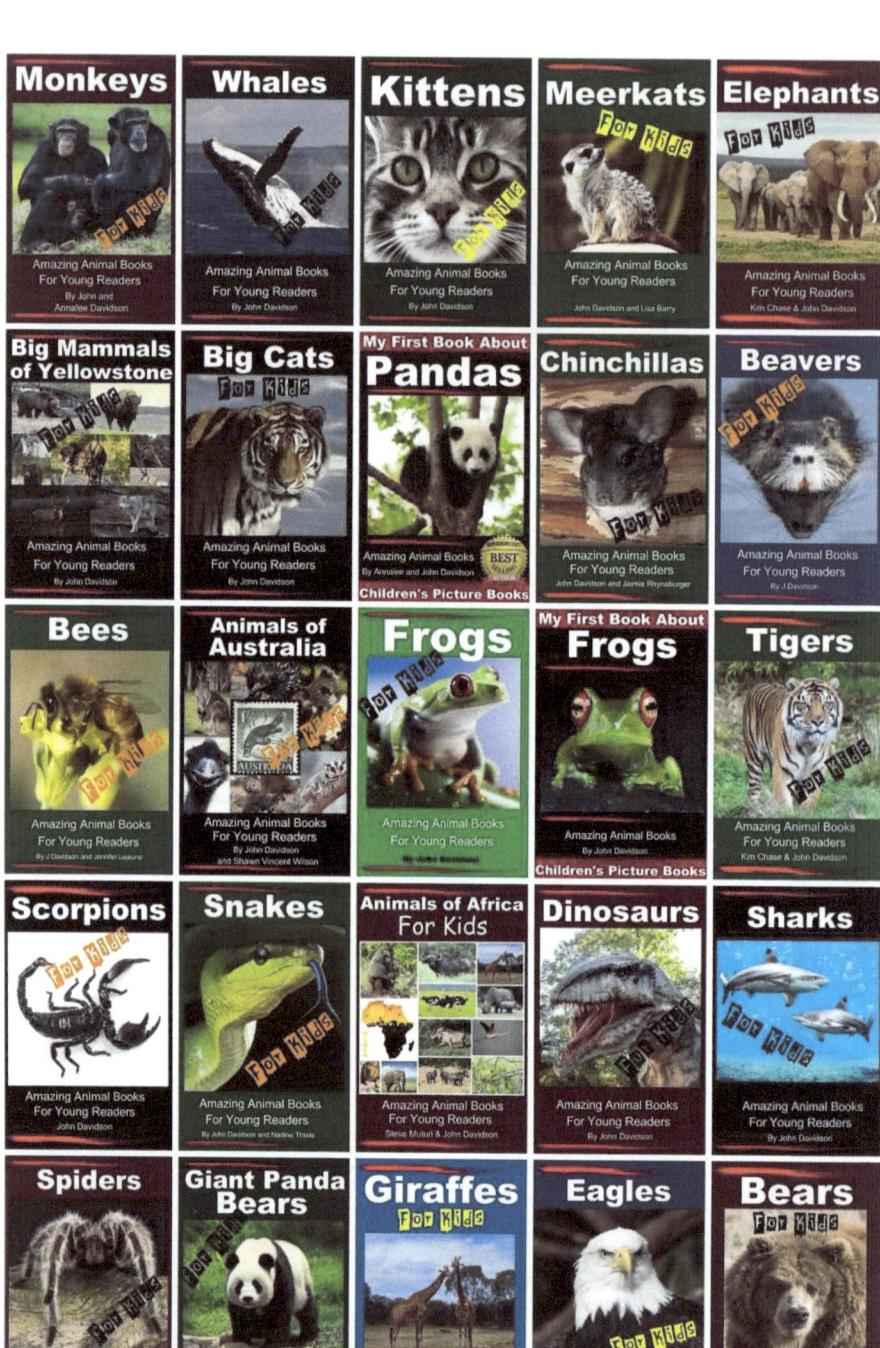

Our books are available at

1. Amazon.com

2. Barnes and Noble

3. Itunes

4. Kobo

5. Smashwords

6. Google Play Books

Download Free Books!
http://MendonCottageBooks.com

Publisher

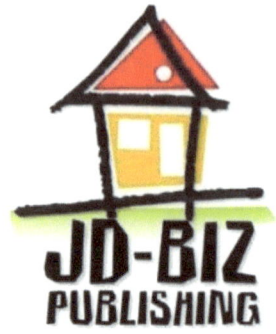

JD-Biz Corp

P O Box 374

Mendon, Utah 84325

http://www.jd-biz.com/

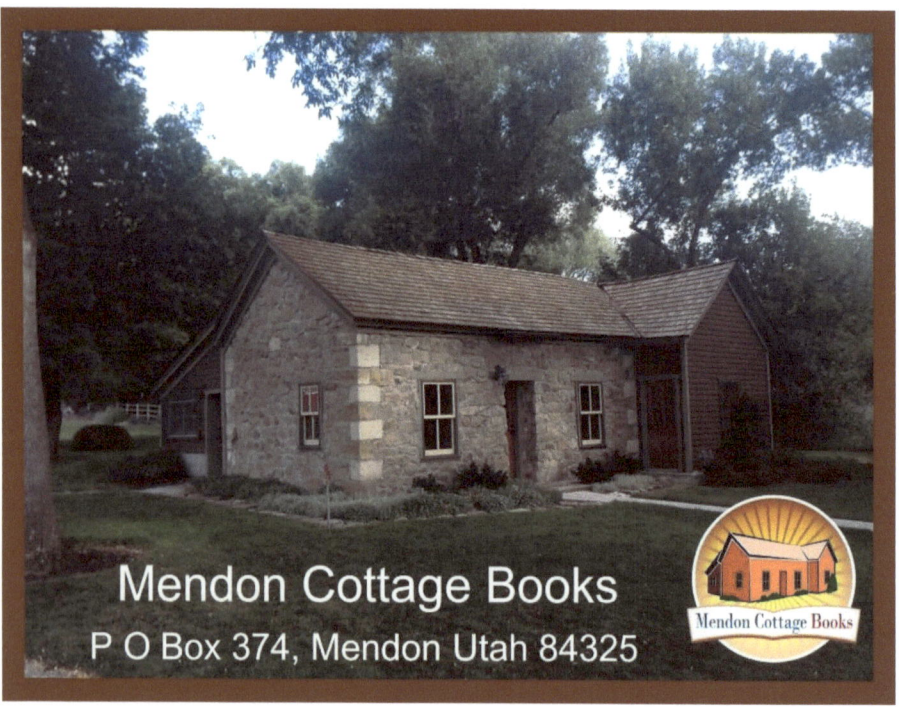

Mendon Cottage Books

P O Box 374, Mendon Utah 84325